As The
Wind Blows

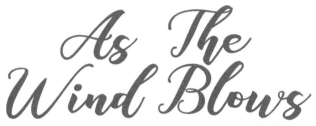

As The Wind Blows

Seven Stories of Women Gaining Strength from Weakness

Shanicka N. Scarbrough, MD

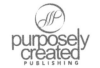

purposely created
PUBLISHING

AS THE WIND BLOWS

Published by Purposely Created Publishing Group™
Copyright © 2017 Shanicka Scarbrough

Printed in the United States of America

ISBN: 978-1-947054-74-5

Special discounts are available on bulk quantity purchases by book clubs, associations, and special interest groups.

For details, please contact
Dr. Shanicka at info@DrShanicka.com.

Therefore I will boast all the more gladly about my weaknesses, so that Christ's power may rest on me. That is why, for Christ's sake, I delight in weaknesses, in insults, in hardships, in persecutions, in difficulties. For when I am weak, then I am strong.

2 Corinthians 12:8-10 (NIV)

To the Overcomers...

"The marvelous richness of human experience would lose something of rewarding joy if there were no limitations to overcome. The hilltop hour would not be half so wonderful if there were no dark valleys to traverse."

—Helen Keller

Table of Contents

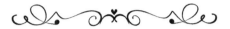

Foreword

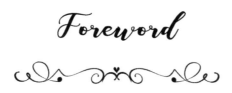

I am honored and excited to be writing the foreword of this book. In meeting Dr. Shanicka over the phone, I think we both realized we had a few things in common. It wasn't just that we are First Ladies of a church (wives of pastors who shepherd churches), but we are women who, contrary to what others may believe, in addition to leadership roles, have the daily struggles of life, including caring for elderly parents and supporting our husbands in ministry, all while having our own dreams and issues to deal with as we take care of so much in a day. Yes, as evidenced in our lives, women can wear many hats. Once we met in person, it was like two little girls found a new friend on the playground of life. We connected through our joys, struggles as women, laughter, and genuine concerns about world issues.

In her chapter, "You Can't Steal My Joy," you will connect with Dr. Shanicka as a young woman developing and working through the struggle of good and evil in a battle for her life. The devil is always on his job to deceive us and play with our emotions and feelings. It's important for us to connect with God, so we know when He's speaking to us versus when the devil is speaking his subtle and sly words of deception. Dr. Shanicka shares very open and transparent accounts of how the enemy desired to destroy her throughout her childhood and well into her adulthood. Thank God, she had enough strength to turn back toward the church and seek help through prayer and the word of God.

If you've experienced any type of hardship or despair, know that there are other powers at work (Ephesians 6:12) and spiritual warfare is needed to fight what you are going through. If you have had some setbacks and are struggling to get back to where you need to be to move forward, then you've picked up the right book to give you hope, joy, and deliverance through the authors' life struggles and stories of redemption through God's presence and His word.

As the women in this book have anchored themselves to truth and peace, you too will need to do the same to make it through a hard time with spiritual attacks. We all need some encouragement from time to time, from real people and real-life situations, so we can say, "I too can overcome!" Reality television shows and the media give us half glimpses of others' glamorous lifestyles and struggles, but they never really tell us how to overcome the drama in a positive and productive way. There's only one way that can happen and one person it can happen through. That's God! Let Dr.

Shanicka and her coauthors take you through their journey and show you how God is waiting to walk you to safety and deliverance when you seek Him first and cry out to Him.

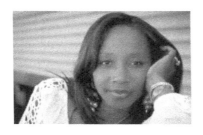

First Lady Dianna L. Lovelace
First Ladies Academy of Sacramento
PO Box 723
Rancho Cordova, CA 95741
Email: FirstLadiesAcademySAC@gmail.com

Preface

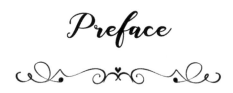

The Sunday before I planned to send in the finished manuscript of this book to our publisher, a pastor from my hometown church, Senior Pastor Jason Reynolds of Emmanuel Baptist Church in San Jose, California, came to preach at our church, BOSS Church of Sacramento, where my husband, Darryl Scarbrough, is the senior pastor. The sermon was powerful and challenged us in ways that only God can through a minister. At the end of the sermon, Pastor Reynolds began to tell a story about trees being cultivated in a man-made environment that was almost identical to our Earth's ecosystem. However, there was one component that was missing, and the lack of this element would lead inevitably to the tree's demise.

The pastor spoke of the University of Arizona's Biosphere 2 project, a facility that was created for the sole purpose of being a research tool for scientists to study the earth's living systems in a controlled environment. One of the most profound discoveries in this research was made during the study of how trees grow. The scientists noticed that the trees growing in the biosphere were growing at a faster rate than if they were in their natural environment. This would have been an awesome discovery had the trees continued to grow to maturity. It came to pass that once the trees reached a certain height, they would start to fall over and die.

After much research into what the difference was between the natural habit and the biosphere, the scientists began to take note of the outer layer of the bark. There they found that in the natural environment, trees grow more slowly because they have to withstand the wind. In order to do so, trees develop an outer layer of what they call stress wood, which is strong and fibrous and helps trees to survive. In the biosphere, without the pressure of the wind blowing, the trees would sprout up but die prematurely, having not developed the strong base of the stress wood that would ensure their survival.

I nearly bolted from my seat as I listened to this pastor sum up the sentiment of this entire book in this real-life parable! As he sat down after closing, I happily shared with him the title of this book that was divinely inspired by his sermon, "As the Wind Blows." Our struggles, our hardships, our heartaches, our troubles, and our tears help strengthen and build up our resilience to adversity. It is in this space where we can truly call out to God, who strengthens our resolve.

This book is a compilation of true stories from women who have chosen to be transparent with themselves and the readers in an effort to show that you are not alone and you too can overcome. Be thankful for the winds that blow in your life, for everything that comes into our lives to oppose us truly only makes us stronger. Hang on, my sister, and watch how God will facilitate your growth and establish a firm foundation on His word right where you are planted. Just let the wind blow.

Chapter 1

The Reason Behind My Smile

Lachelle Evans

❧

*Weeping may endure for a night, but joy
cometh in the morning.*

Psalm 30:5

As a little girl, I was spoiled. Not only that, but I was a middle child, so I always got my way. I thought I was going to continue to be that spoiled little princess who could get whatever she wanted and from whomever she wanted. Ha! That laugh was all on me.

Growing up, I observed how my mom always looked her best whenever she took my brothers and me to the movies, shopping, dinner, or church. My mom always made sure she had money in her purse to get us whatever we wanted. I tried my best to live exactly how she did, to be very independent, to never ask a man for anything, and to work hard for whatever I wanted. Well, that didn't turn out so well. For me, life hasn't been "no crystal stair."

One Sunday morning, my mother became a member of the church. She realized that the life she had been living was not pleasing to God. She went from taking us to different outings, dinners, shows, and birthday parties to going to church all day, every day, in addition to the traditional Sundays—all because she had decided to give her life to Christ. What did that mean for her children? For me, it meant I became the little sanctified girl who could go nowhere but school, church, and home. No movies, no pajama parties, no birthday parties—all of the things that I had grown accustomed to!

Church became a second home to my brothers and me. Because we were at church so much and had to obey my mother's new way of living, I decided to join as well. I became an usher on the usher board, and attended Sunday school and youth services. At the time, it was wonderful because we met some awesome people who became like family. But my mother had always been the outgoing mommy who loved to do fun stuff. When she turned her life over to Christ, we all had to make that change to what seemed like a mundane life.

As the years went on, my siblings and I became frustrated. Mom was strict about everything. I stopped feeling important to anyone and felt like no one was paying attention to me, so I became rebellious. I began talking back and not doing so well in school. I began sneaking in and out of the house to be with my friends. And guess what? You got it! All that sneaking and hanging out got me pregnant at the age of fifteen.

I didn't know what to do. I felt very alone and insecure about myself. My self-esteem and popularity in school suffered because of the pregnancy. Where had all of those friends I was sneaking out to hang out with gone?

When I worked up the courage to tell my mother, as you can probably guess, she was very disappointed in me. She often yelled at me because she was embarrassed by the snickers and rumors about me at church. I was so ashamed that I wouldn't step foot through the doors of the church, the one place where there was supposed to be comfort instead of judgment.

To add salt to the wound, three months after the birth of my first son, I found out I was pregnant again! Here I was, sixteen years old, carrying a second child. And I was still a child myself. My parents couldn't hide their disappointment. This pushed me further into isolation. I couldn't do anything, I couldn't go anywhere—I felt trapped.

Every now and then, I would go outside with both babies, my daughter in the stroller and my son walking beside me. It seemed I only got attention from older men, which made me feel more mature, important, and sexy. I didn't date any of the guys, I just loved the attention they gave me. They made me feel validated because the little popular girl and daddy's princess wasn't feeling so popular anymore. My relationship with the babies' father was unstable, and he was in and out of our lives. I was in love with my babies, but I felt so isolated being the only teenager on my block who had babies. I knew something had to change—life had to change.

One hot summer night, as I was walking home, I heard a car horn honking. When I turned around to investigate, I saw a gold Cadillac with tinted windows. The driver, a caramel-skinned guy, was waving his hand for me to come across the street to join him. He was fine! I sashayed my way over to him, being sure he got a close look at my oiled-down bowed legs peeking out from under my black mini-skirt. I had on a red blouse with red and white ankle socks and white-girl gym shoes that completed my sexy, flirty look. As I approached him, I could smell his enticing cologne, and I could see the shine of his fresh curls, thanks to the curl activator spray. He was blinged out and had a smile that was calling me closer to him.

He casually stated, "Get in."

Cautiously, I said, "No, why? I have my babies with me. I'm fine right here. What's up?"

"You're beautiful with an amazing smile, white teeth sparkling."

I chuckled like I had won the lottery. I was tingling on the inside and felt my heart beating fast in my chest. I grasped my son's hands tightly while my daughter slept quietly in her stroller. The conversation went on easily from there, and we laughed and talked for almost an hour.

My kids were beginning to get restless, and he noted that we had been out there long enough, so he offered to take us home. For some strange reason, I felt so secure with this guy. After dropping us off, he asked me out. I gladly accepted.

The following week, on a sunny Saturday morning, he took me out to one of the neighborhood's popular breakfast spots. While we were laughing and joking around, I noticed there were many women who were calling him "Daddy," and strangely, they were staring at me up and down.

I asked him, "Why are your friends looking at me like that?"

He smiled and said, "Baby girl, don't worry about them. They want what you have."

Oooohhh, he was slick!

"Smooth operator you are," I said.

"Oh no, baby girl, not I," he responded, with laughter in his soft voice.

He gently grasped my hands and placed his warm wet lips on top of my hands with a kiss and stated he wanted me to "be his main squeeze."

I accepted with the biggest smile, not even second-guessing what he meant by "main squeeze." I finally had a boyfriend, someone who was giving me the attention I needed!

He said I was his and that I could have whatever I wanted. He was playing right into the spoiled girl ego from my childhood. He promised to take good care of me and my babies.

Then he said it was getting late and he had to hurry to get to work before the rain started. With sadness, I asked when I would see him again.

"Real soon, sweetheart, okay?" he said.

"If you say so," I said.

He looked at me with anger and said in a deep, Barry White voice, "What you say? I see Imma have to teach you how to talk to Daddy with respect!"

I chuckled and thought nothing of what he was saying and looked the other way. After he paid for the food, the same ladies from earlier came back to the restaurant. They seemed kind of worried, as if they were going to get in trouble. Needless to say, he left the table and went to talk to them. I just sat at the table with fire in my eyes, waiting and watching until he was finished.

"Those ladies really like touching on you, huh?" I said.

Of course, he responded, "They ain't nobody, just ladies looking for attention. You all I want, baby girl, but I have a lot of lady friends, okay!"

He grabbed my hand and pulled me closer to him. The smell of his cologne began to take over my body with a tingling sensation. He kissed me on top of my forehead, slowly. He followed with slow kisses on my jaws and behind my ears, whispering, "Are you ready for a man like me in your life?"

My eyes blinked softly after every kiss. I was melting inside, my hormones taking over. I didn't know what to think or say, but out of nowhere, I said, "Ready for what?"

The kisses stopped. "I need to take you home now."

"Why?" I asked.

"I told you earlier I have to go to work. I have things to do."

At that moment, I felt cold and alone, as if I had done something wrong. He waved at the waitress to come get the money.

We exited the door of the restaurant into the pouring rain. As we ran to the car, he shielded me with some newspapers from the newsstand outside the restaurant. Once we made it to the car, both soaking wet, he began to wipe the water from the pouring rain off my face with his gentle hands, smelling like maple syrup. Every time he touched me, my body had a mind of its own.

When we arrived at my house, he opened the glove compartment and handed me a white envelope, telling me to get the kids and myself something. He was going out of town, so this would hold me over until he got back.

He grasped my hands to move closer to him. Our lips touched, and there it was again—kissing like never before. So intense, full of wetness and passion. He began rubbing on me and caressing my shoulders while he gently placed his other hand on my face. With my eyes closed, all I could hear was him saying "baby girl" in that soft, Babyface voice. Then he said we had to stop because he had to go but to make some time for "Daddy" once he got back. He got out of the car to open the door for me, and as he looked up to the skies, he laughed and said, "See what kissing you does?"

I looked up at the clear sky, the clouds all puffy and white. He began singing "I Can See Clearly Now," an old-school song by Johnny Nash. We both laughed and looked at each other with glazing desire. I had to stop for a moment and realize that this man only had eyes for me and that I was his girlfriend. In that moment, I felt like I was important to him.

When I walked into the house, I heard my mom talking on the phone saying, "Lord, I have to go to church, this child needs to get home to these kids."

I called out, "Hey Mom, I'm home!"

She looked at me and said, "Where have you been?"

"Nowhere, Mommy, I was down the street talking to one of my friends."

Oh boy, my mom gave me that look saying I needed to stop lying and take my kids with me the next time I left because she wasn't no built-in babysitter. She walked to her bedroom and slammed the door. I stomped off and tried to slam my bedroom door, but it didn't work because my mother was right there in the doorway, saying, "I wish you would slam a door in my house!"

Once my mom went into her bedroom, I ripped open the envelope. There was a letter. I unfolded the paper and out dropped four one hundred dollar bills. My eyes went to the letter, which read, *I have a beeper for you to pick up. Here's the address and beeper number and our communication numbers are 1234 I miss you and 1233 Meet me outside.* I started dancing.

The next morning, I quickly got dressed and headed out, leaving my babies to sleep in the bed while my mom watched over them. I made a note to myself not to forget to get them something.

Weeks went by, and I was missing him so much. Then, I heard a beep! I picked up the beeper and saw the numbers 1234. Wow, was I excited. Then it beeped again: 1233. I ran out the door, and there he was.

"I just had to see your beautiful face and give you these roses."

"Oh my," I said, feeling loved and missed by this handsome Babyface-looking guy.

He said he wanted to meet later, after he had unpacked.

Later that night, my daughter and I were heading home from a birthday party. As I walked down the main street to get home, I saw the neighborhood barber who cut my son's hair.

"Hey, be careful going home and don't forget your son's appointment tomorrow!" he said.

"Okay," I said with a smile, "I won't!"

Minutes later, I heard a horn honking at me. I watched as the car pulled up. It was my guy, looking at me with fire in his eyes. He told me to get in the car. As soon as I got in the car, he began yelling and cursing at me, demanding the reason why I hadn't answer his beep. He'd been sitting in the alley all that time.

"I honestly didn't hear the beep, baby."

"Of course not because you're showing your body and smiling, laughing with him while I'm waiting for you. You're acting like a ho!"

I started crying. "Why are you talking to me like this?"

"Shut up!"

He slapped me across the face. I clutched my baby and held my face with disbelief. I had done nothing wrong. He began to drive off, speeding faster at every curve. My baby was crying, and I was crying, pleading for him to slow down and take me home. He stopped the car in the middle of the street. I reached to open the door, but he locked the door from his side.

"Bitch, you're not going nowhere."

He slapped me again and told me to shut up my daughter. I continued to cry and scream for him to let me out. He parked at a house and told me to get out. I didn't know where I was.

I got out crying, my nose running, my baby crying and screaming. He told me to put my baby in the car because it had started to rain. I did not want to let my daughter go. I was terrified and scared. But I didn't want her getting sick, so I placed my baby in the back seat and stood outside of the car.

Out of nowhere, I felt another slap across my face. And then again and again and again, until my nose bled. He didn't stop. I screamed for him to stop hitting me, as blood ran down my shirt.

He dragged me by my hair from the car, yelling at me. I was screaming for my baby. Once he lost his hold on me, I tried to run my hardest to the car to get my baby, but he ran after me.

"Don't you dare!" he said. "Let's go in the house now."

I held my baby in my arms as tight as I could. I couldn't break away from him as he pulled me up the stairs.

"I just want to go," I said.

He pointed a gun in my face and said, "You and your baby are not going anywhere."

He grabbed me and beat me with the pistol while my baby was lying on the bed crying and screaming her lungs out.

I yelled to him, "Don't kill me, please, my baby needs me, please! Please! I'm sorry!"

He said, "Now you are going to make me happy and give me what I want."

He lay on top of me, my head moving back and forth, saying "No, don't kiss me, don't do this, let me go! My baby, my baby."

Slap. He snatched my blouse open, ripped my underwear, and began to have sex with me, saying I better shut up and enjoy it. He said he owned me. I was unable to breathe. I felt it was over. He was going to kill me and my baby.

After he got off me, I turned and grabbed my baby and just lay there, too scared to move. I couldn't believe what had just happened. He got up, locked the door, and said not to move until he got some sleep. He took out the bullets from the gun and placed the gun in between us.

The whole night, I stayed up trying to figure out what I had done wrong to this man. I thought to myself, if this is liking or loving someone, this is not for me. I thought about how I was going to get my baby and me out of the house, not knowing what would happen if he caught us. I just had to get out.

There was a knock on the door. When he opened the door, I heard him say he'd be down soon. He left without locking the door, his gun still on the bed. I got up slowly, in severe pain, bloody and sore. I grabbed my baby girl and slowly walked out of the bedroom. The coast was clear. I opened the front door and ran down the street as fast as I could with my baby in my arms. I ran barefoot all the way home, never looking back. I was running for our lives.

When I arrived home, I ran to my bedroom and closed the door. Wet, I got under the covers, holding my baby tight. My heart was beating fast and my eyes were racing back and forth. I thought he was going to come to the house and kill us!

The next morning, I felt hopeless, afraid, and worthless. I didn't know what to do. I was scared to tell my mom, scared to talk to anyone. I finally got up to feed my baby, wash her, and put her to sleep. I looked at myself in the mirror and broke down in tears. I got in the shower and let the water run all over my body, cleaning the blood off me. My face and body were so sore and bruised up. I think I ran that shower for hours, scrubbing my entire body over and over again.

When I got out of the shower, I suddenly heard a voice say, *My child, you have forsaken me, I haven't forsaken you. You are still my child, I will take care of you, but first you have to repent and don't get revenge!*

Not knowing what to think or do besides cry, I thought of taking revenge and all the ways I could get him back. Not once did I think to tell my mom or call the police. I just kept that dark secret to myself, even after my mother asked me what was wrong and if there was something I needed to talk about. I was ashamed, hurt, and embarrassed because I felt I had no one to blame but myself.

The next day, I went to a routine checkup with the doctor. On my way home, I began to cry to God, saying, *I'm sorry, Lord, please, please forgive me.* I asked Him, *why me? Why did this happen to me? I thought he loved me.*

That little voice spoke to me again. *You don't even love yourself! You have to love you!*

At that moment, I began walking faster toward my house. I walked in, looked at my mom, ran to her, gave her the biggest hug, and began to cry on her shoulders.

"Mom, will I ever be somebody?"

My mom looked at me and said, "You are somebody. You're my daughter and your children's mother and God's child. Honey, God forgives us of our sins. He loves you, that's all you need."

I didn't know if my mom knew or not, but at that moment, I felt loved!

The next day, I ran into my friend from the barbershop. He told me "your guy" and some of those girls had gotten locked up for drugs and prostitution. He said they had some long years of time to do. What! I felt relieved and sick to my stomach all at once. I couldn't believe I had been with a pimp! Looking back, there were signs—ladies, money, trips out of town, and expensive cars.

On my way home from the store, there was that voice again: *Don't weep for him, my child, but rejoice in me for I haven't given up on you.*

I began crying tears of relief. I went into the bathroom and looked in the mirror. I told myself, I love you! You're beautiful with an amazing smile. I stopped looking back and started moving forward. I gained a whole new level of respect for myself and started loving myself first. I realized that I am somebody, that God kept me here not only for my babies and my mom, but to help someone else, to motivate others. This is the reason for my smile—to help encourage, empower, and motivate women of all ages who have low self-esteem, to let you know you are somebody.

Repeat to yourself: I'm somebody! I'm an overcomer! I'm a child of God! I'm me! I'm beautiful! I'm here!

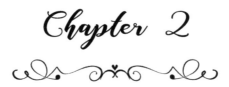

Chapter 2

My Destiny

Timika Lucas

We glory in tribulations also: knowing that tribulation worketh patience;

And patience, experience; and experience, hope.

Romans 5:3-4

*A*s I walked down the hall toward my room, with tears running down my face, I felt helpless. Seeing all the moms leave with their babies and excited to get home was overwhelming. The thought of leaving my baby was devastating.

When I found out I was pregnant for the third time, I was excited—not only because I was having another baby, but because this time it was different. I was older, more financially stable, and overall in a better place. My daughters were extremely excited about having another brother or sister.

My pregnancy was, initially, as normal as the first two. Morning sickness was alive and well. I would get nauseous at the drop of a hat. It got so bad that sometimes the mere task of driving would make my head spin. Every doctor's visit was fine. No concerns or issues arose, and the baby's heartbeat was strong. The baby was growing at a normal rate, and I was gaining a lot of weight. During my last doctor's visit prior to giving birth, we found out I was having another girl. Having two girls already, my boyfriend was a little disappointed that it wasn't a boy, but he was excited all the same. Little did we know, the last stretch of this pregnancy would be nothing like my first two pregnancies.

Monday, August 6, 2007, started like any other day. I woke up, got in the shower, and started to get ready for work. As I was dressing, I noticed that my underwear was wet, as if I had urinated on myself. I felt a little strange but shrugged it off. I changed my underwear and continued to get dressed. As I felt fluid leave my body again, I knew I couldn't be peeing on myself. It wasn't the normal warm, thin, free-flowing fluid that one feels. It was warm, with a thicker consistency, and it dripped out of me like molasses from a tree. I called the doctor's office and spoke to a nurse. She asked me how often I was wetting myself. When I told her it seemed like every five minutes, she told me my water bag may be leaking and that I should go to the emergency room.

Now I had experienced my water bag leaking with my second child. But this was different. I knew it was serious when I was told to go to the ER. When I arrived at the emergency room and told the triage nurse why I was there, I was immediately put in a wheelchair and taken to an exam room. I was given a gown and was asked to undress. As I sat on the cold wrinkled sheets on the flat mattress of the gurney, I said a small prayer. *Please, Lord, let my baby be okay.* While waiting on the doctor to come in, I was a little nervous, given that I had been told that I had a leaking water bag, which I knew wasn't good because I was only twenty-three weeks, yet I was not fearful.

I wasn't fearful, not because the situation didn't call for it, but because I had been working in a hospital for nine years. This type of environment was normal for me to be in. But the moment the doctor came in, I became anxious. She did the usual pelvic exam to confirm that my water bag was thinning. After a series of tests were performed, the doctor told me that I would be staying. The thought of not going home was concerning. I thought that I would be pumped full of fluids for a couple of days, my water bag would replenish itself, and I would be able to go home. At the time, I didn't know—but I would later find out—that I was diagnosed with PROM, premature rupture of membranes.

After spending more than enough time in the emergency room, I was transferred to a room on the maternity floor. It was a little weird for me because for nine years, I was the one who transported patients around the hospital via a wheelchair or stretcher, and here I was—a patient being transported to Labor and Delivery at twenty-three weeks pregnant. Even at that moment, as I was wheeled through the halls of the hospital, I still hadn't consciously grasped the seriousness of the events that were unfolding.

The first twenty-four hours in the hospital were scary. There were nurses coming in and out, taking my vitals and drawing my blood. I felt like a human pincushion. Even though I was given some information as to what was going on, there were still questions that I had, and panic was slowly rearing its ugly head.

Finally, a maternal fetal doctor, who specializes in high-risk pregnancies, came in. As I lay there anticipating the words that would come out of his mouth, he looked over my chart, pulled up a chair next to my bed, and said, "At this point in your pregnancy, if you were to deliver today, your baby would not be viable. A baby born before twenty-four weeks is considered non-viable. If this happens, do you want us to do anything and everything we can to save your baby?"

"Of course," I replied.

He continued to explain to me the plan of treatment and what I could expect.

The plan was to pump me full of liquids, just as I thought, to see if that would replenish the fluid in my water bag and to keep the baby in the womb as long as they possibly could. This meant that I could be there for days, weeks, or months. I didn't know what to think. One minute I was in the comfort of my own home, and the next I was in the hospital fighting for my baby's life. After the doctor left, the nurse walked in with a needle longer than my arm. She must have seen the bewildered look on my face because she immediately started explaining what it was for. It was a medication to strengthen my baby's lungs. The catch was, it had to be administered in my butt. I was given more medicine to keep me from going into labor and given plenty of water to drink.

I wasn't allowed to move. I could not leave my bed for anything. I couldn't even get up to go to the bathroom to bathe or release myself. I had to have a sponge bath in the bed and use a bedpan to urinate in. I had never felt so vulnerable and helpless in my life. There are many times when I wished I could just lie in the bed all day, but to be forced to do so and be dependent on others to do the simplest acts devastated me. I was afraid that I wouldn't be able to hold her long enough to where she would be developed enough to thrive outside the womb. There was nothing I could do but hope and pray that my baby stay put. I often lay in my hospital bed wondering what I had done to cause this. Was it something I ate? Should I have continued to work? Was I doing too much?

Blaming myself was the only logical thing I could do. God gave me one task, to provide a safe and healthy womb for my child to grow, and I couldn't do that. I had two other children, six and eight years old, who I had to take care of. Could I have overexerted myself and not known it? No one could tell me how or why this had happened. The only reply I got was, "sometimes things like this happen."

That may be true, but all I could think was why did it have to happen to me?

For sixteen days, from August 6 to August 22, I lay in bed twenty-four hours a day. I missed my daughters' first day of school and my nephew's ninth birthday. Life was going on around me as I lay stagnant in a hospital room, hoping I would not go into labor. Emotionally, I was numb to the situation. I decided to take one day at a time and do what I could to keep her in the womb. At one point, a nurse said to me, "You are taking this whole situation well compared to other patients I have had in similar circumstances. By day three, moms are pulling their hair out from not being able to move around."

A long time ago, I learned not to stress about things I have no control over. Stressing myself out would only make the situation worse, not only for me but also for my daughter. I know what you're thinking—how could you not be freaking out being that you thought you may lose your child? How could I? Stressing and worrying about it would have caused physical stress to my body and my baby. I didn't want to diminish the chances of her being as healthy as she possibly could. At that point, the reality of the situation had not fully hit me yet. I knew what was going on and what the outcome could be, but the severity of the situation had not manifested itself yet.

On the morning of August 21, I was informed that a C-section would be performed the next day. After sixteen days in the hospital, the doctors determined that no matter how much water I drank, my water bag was not refilling. Since I had made it to twenty-five weeks, my daughter had a chance to survive.

August 22 changed the course of my life forever. I spiked a fever, so I was told that a C-section would be performed that morning. At around 11:15 a.m., at almost twenty-six weeks, my Destiny was born. I would later learn that the cause of her being born prematurely was due to a diagnosis of probable chorioamnionitis, inflammation of my amniotic fluid from a bacterial infection. One pound, nine ounces, and nine inches long, Destiny was whisked off to the neonatal intensive care unit (NICU). But before she was taken from the room, I could see her, and all I saw were big, hazel brown eyes staring at me. Even then, she was looking for her mom.

For the first twenty-four hours, I lay in bed resting from my C-section, wondering how my baby was doing and what was happening to her. Many thoughts were going through my head. Will she be all right? Will she have any long-lasting mental or physical problems? Will she survive? Throughout the day, as the nurses came in and out of my room, I continued to ask how my daughter was doing and when I would be able to see her. The nurses kept reassuring me that my baby was in the best hands and I should get some sleep. But how could I sleep when my daughter was fighting for her life? Not knowing was the worst feeling I ever had.

The next morning, I was encouraged to get up and walk to help strengthen my muscles. As I walked the halls of the maternity floor, gripping the cold, colorful concrete walls for support, I saw the new moms with their babies, making me miss Destiny even more. Even though she wasn't that far away, she wasn't there with me. Although Destiny was my third child, it had been six years since I had had a baby around. It was important that we had those initial mom–baby bonding moments. Holding her close to me, inhaling that newborn baby smell, watching her as she slept, and seeing the different facial expressions appear on her face as she dreamed her first dreams are moments that were taken away from me, and I could never get them back.

Walking to the neonatal intensive care unit was exciting and scary at the same time. Exciting because I was going to see my baby up close for the first time. Scary because I didn't know what to expect when I saw her. The five-minute walk felt like forever. With every step I took toward the nursery, the more nervous I became. As I approached the nurses' station, I paused, said a short prayer, and prepared myself for what I might see. As I stood at the door of the NICU pod, a feeling of anxiety, excitement, and fear overcame me, and at that moment, I was ready to see my Destiny.

I entered the pod, and in the first incubator I saw was my baby. There she lay, her tiny little body with a tube in her nose for feeding because of her inability to suck, swallow, and breathe at the same time, one in her naval (an umbilical catheter) to administer medication and fluids, and one in her chest (a broviac catheter) to administer medication and draw blood. Overwhelmed, excited, scared, anxious, and awestruck—I was hit with many emotions at once— the tears started to flow. I was so happy to see my baby. I wanted to touch her, but because her nervous system was so underdeveloped, I wasn't allowed to as it may have caused overstimulation.

My daughter was nine inches—about the length of my hand. As I sat next to her bed, watching her breathe, in awe of the tiny diaper that she wore, the urge to hold my child was so overwhelming that I couldn't do anything but cry. I sat next to her for as long as the nurses allowed, through shift changes and doctors' rounds. After several hours, I had to return to my room, as I needed to not only get some rest but to also have my nurses make sure I was okay. But as long as my child was in the NICU, I wasn't okay. As I took that long walk back to my room, again gripping the cold walls for support, I anticipated seeing my daughter the next day.

By day two, I had regained a little strength, and the time it took me to get to the NICU was a little shorter. Again, I sat by her side, watching the ventilator help her take each breath. The nurses gave her medication to help increase her brain activity, strengthen her lungs, and feed her the milk that I had pumped that morning to help her thrive. I listened as the doctors rounded on her, as the attendings and residents conversed about her daily progress and plans of action. Having a baby in the NICU, you come to realize that nothing happens overnight, and there's a process for everything. You consistently hear "we just have to wait and see" for medications to work or for procedures to correct an issue. You learn that you must depend on time, an unknown, unspecified, intangible concept that determines the fate of your child.

On day three, August 25, my last day as a patient, I went to visit my baby again. As I sat there watching her, my mind began to wander back to the question that I had asked myself repeatedly: why did this happen to her? What could I have done to cause a different outcome? What did I do to cause my water bag to leak? The answers to some of these questions would never be answered.

When the time came for me to leave the NICU, something happened that forever will be ingrained in my mind. My baby started to cry. And although her tear ducts were not producing tears and her vocal cords were not strong enough to produce a sound, the expression on her face said it all. Unable to perform the simplest act of motherhood, pick my baby up and console her, all I could do was stand there and watch her. At that moment, the reality of everything that I had gone through for the past nineteen days hit me like a ton of bricks, and I started to cry.

As I walked down the hall toward my room, with tears running down my face, I felt helpless. Seeing all the moms leaving with their babies and excited to get home was overwhelming. The thought of leaving my baby was devastating. I felt worthless and empty, joined by a sense of failure. I had held my baby for twenty-five weeks and had failed to keep her healthy. Now I was being punished for my failure. I wouldn't be able to enjoy bringing my baby home. I would miss the joys and looks of happiness and excitement on my girls' faces as they saw their sister for the first time. My punishment was watching my daughter fight for her life for the next ninety days and be reminded of how I had failed her.

But oh, for the love of God and the many blessings that He bestows upon His children daily. My blessing was seeing my daughter fight and become stronger with each breath she took, unlike so many other mothers and fathers who don't get that opportunity.

On November 23, 2007, Destiny was discharged from the hospital. I was finally able to share in the excitement that I had seen the other mothers express three months before. Even though she came home with an oxygen tank, a pulse oximeter, a heart monitor, and a feeding tube, she still made it. According to preemiesurvival.com, less than 1 percent of babies in the country are born before twenty-eight weeks, and there is a 50 percent survival rate with a greater risk of severe disability and lower cognitive function results for boys compared with girls. My daughter spent the first year seeing speech therapists, physical therapists, occupational therapists, and doctors. She was weaned off oxygen by that December, and I taught her how to drink from a bottle. Cognitive and neurological impairment is common at school age amongst extremely preterm children. Now, at nine years old, Destiny shows some cognitive impairment in school as she progresses through each grade, but with extra help from teachers, she's showing promise.

For years after Destiny was born, I wanted to have other children, but I was afraid to. I was afraid of having to go through another premature birth. No matter how often I got the baby blues and was assured by my doctor of the minimal chances of it happening again, the fear was still there. What I learned from this experience is that no matter how much you try to do what's right, make the right decisions, follow all the doctor's recommendations, and eat right, there's nothing that can prevent circumstances from occurring.

I'm a strong believer that everything happens for a reason, and we may not understand it or like it, but we try to learn from our experiences and encourage others who may be going through the same situation. When all seems lost or incomprehensible, the best thing you should do is trust that in all things, God works for the good of those who love him, who have been called according to his purpose (Romans 8:28 NIV).

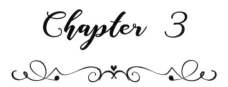

Chapter 3

Overcoming Infertility

Dr. Jerisa Berry

*Let not your heart be troubled,
neither let it be afraid.*

John 14-27

It's an airy feeling when you first see a fertility specialist and you hear the words, "I'm sorry, but you two have less than a 10 percent chance of conceiving naturally." In your youth, you don't imagine that on your path to becoming successful and finding true love that this will be your reality. I was thirty-eight years old when I visited the specialist, but many women are forced to take those steps at a younger age, and unfortunately, may not realize until it's too late that the chances of success are slim.

Fibroid surgery, miscarriages, in vitro fertilization, and countless ultrasounds, shots, blood work, and medications can weigh heavily on women experiencing issues conceiving naturally. According to the American Society of Reproductive Medicine (2012) and the National Survey of Family Growth (2010), over seven million women in the United States have undergone some variant of assisted fertilization techniques to help them become a mother. I am one in seven million in America. How did this happen to me? And excuse my French, but who the heck thinks about fertility when they are young, single, and building a career?

How many single ladies are not mothers because they choose to wait for the right partner? The numbers are astounding: according to the US Census Bureau (2016) and America's Family and Living Arrangements Table (2015),

50 percent of the US population is single. I was single and waiting for my handsome knight in shining armor until I was thirty-five years old. As a physician, it was a sacrifice to reach my life goal of becoming a doctor. I had it all together. I was successful. I have no regrets and certainly had my share of fun, but it wasn't until I met my husband that I found real love—the love that brings to life, "Good things come to those who wait." Together, we decided to wait a little before parenthood, to experience each other, to travel, to goal set and plan. We thought we had time. But years later, we experienced our share of difficulties trying to expand our family.

For almost three years, my husband and I went to countless doctors' appointments. I took several medications, and had to have shots, ultrasounds, and surgeries. It was a very trying time. There were aspects of both of our health that we needed to correct. For example, I was deficient in Vitamin D and also dealt with the most stressing health issue: fibroids. Fibroids are tumors on a mission! They are considered benign, but they can wreak havoc on many women. Initially, I had several small ones, which don't usually pose a major problem, yet a repeat ultrasound one year after the discovery of those small fibroids showed I had a new one inside my uterus that required surgery in order to improve my success rate. This was completely unexpected, as less than one year before, I hadn't needed surgery.

What do you do when life takes you on an unexpected path, one that can be scary and life threatening? At first, I was discouraged, and I didn't want to have the surgery. I told the doctor "no." But within a week, I came to my senses and realized that the surgery was necessary. So despite my surprise, denial, and dismay, I agreed to surgery. Sometimes there's no way to go through life than to just go through it and move forward. That's what I did. Without knowing the outcome. Without knowing the benefit. But knowing that those were steps I had to take in order to try my best.

Surgery went well, and my husband and I continued on our path to parenthood with the help of assisted fertilization. We were ready. We had prayed. And yet again, we were hit with another setback. At this point, I thought, "Really, God? Really." We had to cancel an IVF cycle because of an ovarian cyst that came out of nowhere! I had no prior knowledge of an ovarian cyst, so why now? The doctors said it was due to the medication, and there was nothing we could do but wait and allow it to naturally resorb, which it did in less than two months. But two months feels like one year when you are hoping to conceive after two years of trying.

My revelation during those two months was that as much as we try to control our life, when we believe in a higher power and ask Him to be in control, we relinquish our own. So as much as you plan, plot, and organize, ultimately, your life is constructed by God. This can be both scary and relieving at the same time. Scary because you feel you work so hard and deserve your want when you want it, but relieving because God can do things so much better than you can ever even imagine.

After the cyst absorbed, we were ready and excited once more. We went through another IVF, during which my fibroids grew larger from the medications. Thankfully, I had embryos, but because my fibroids were back—with a vengeance I might add—even after surgery, we decided to go another route in our quest for parenting.

There are some women who have difficulties getting pregnant. There are others who have difficulty maintaining a pregnancy. To our surprise, we were happy when we became pregnant after our second IVF treatment, but it was short-lived, unviable, and resulted in a miscarriage. Just when you think you've overcome, BOOM! Another trial. But trials come to test our patience, our faith. Through it all, we maintained hope, maintained our praise, and we found light in offering other women a solution to understand their biological clock.

For those of you who haven't experienced a miscarriage and the devastation it causes, let me give some insight. My experience wasn't as bad as some women because my pregnancy was a surprise in itself. But for many women, a part of them dies. How can you love what you've never seen? And how can you be so hurt? A miscarriage causes a loss that continues long after the passage. Not only because of the loss of the fetus, but also because of the doubt it brings upon you about your potential inability to carry a child or become a mother. This is what makes many women fearful of even attempting another pregnancy. You remember how you felt when you failed a class in school? Well, it's not like that. It's much worse. Failing at becoming a mom and getting through pregnancy takes a big chunk out of your confidence level, your security, and your worthiness. For months, and for some women, years, you feel the void of the loss. It takes special coping skills to handle all the emotions that come with having a miscarriage. Many of these coping mechanisms are not necessarily innate within us. For me, I was able to manage my emotions from my miscarriage much better than my emotions from our failed IVF cycle.

How did I overcome all the negative emotions? I had to remember that my wants do not necessarily match my needs. This is an important concept to grasp. Without thinking about life this way, you will always be depressed when things do not go as you planned. The other thought that helped me was realizing that in parenting, although you birth a child into this world, they ultimately still do not *really* belong to you. As a child grows and moves out of a home, they are released into the world, in a sense. They are always your loved one, but their life belongs to a higher power. Their steps are ordered, except when guided under their own selfish will. This helps many parents who have unfortunately lost a child. The same concept applies to those who do not yet have children. I realized that my life could not depend on whether I became a mother or not. I needed to still go ahead and live my life as it is presently.

Tomorrow is not promised. This can be such a cliché, but as an emergency room physician, I see and manage death all the time. Because of this experience, I know first-hand that so many people live for tomorrow, not realizing that today could very well be their last. Thus, on my doubtful days, I lean on this thought: we need to live for today! This is another way I overcome difficult times.

When becoming an ER doctor, while we learn biology, we learn nothing about the woman's biological clock. For many women, becoming a mother while young will not be difficult. Infertility is not only a problem of women in their thirties; the issues could have begun in their twenties but they hadn't become aware of it because they weren't ready to start a family at that time. Imagine all the twenty-something-year-olds who are single and living their life, but are unaware where they stand on the biological clock. Yes, as a woman ages, her fertility declines, but fertility actually starts to decline once a woman first menstruates. It's important to become aware of potential problems early, as this helps single women, career-minded women, and waiting women understand their fertility.

It was a tough ride to overcome infertility—a very tough ride. But I am so thankful for the way not just science but caring women who volunteer to be surrogates have revolutionized the ability for desiring couples to have the dream of family become a reality. There's nothing wrong with waiting, but it's the knowledge you possess during the wait that can help bring peace later.

Now, I'm so happy that I see the benefit in my trials and how I can reach back and help other women who are not necessarily considering their fertility during their single years. Now, I encourage and inspire other women who are building their career and delaying motherhood to be mindful of securing their fertility in the meantime. You may hit rock bottom, and you may want to give up, but God certainly will turn your test into a testimony and surround you with believers. Stay faithful through the storm and watch what God will do.

Chapter 4

Adversity

Dr. Tamika Bush

Rejoicing in hope; patient in tribulation;
continuing instant in prayer.

Romans 12:12

Growing up in Detroit, I could have easily gotten involved in the wrong circle of crime, drug abuse, and teen pregnancy. But the foundation and strong core values instilled in me by my mother helped shape me into the woman you see today. Each day, my mother instilled in me the importance of strength, hard work, perseverance, and the importance of being prayerful and putting God first in my life. A Bible verse that always speaks to my heart and is my foundation for my strength as a single mom is Proverbs 22:6 (ERV): "Teach children in a way that fits their needs, and even when they are old, they will not leave the right path."

My life started off as typical. I was born to a middle class family living on the West Side of Detroit. But as I came of age, things became more and more difficult for me. When I was in middle school, my parents began to have difficulties in their relationship. This was an awkward time for me because I was starting to become a young woman and attempting to find myself. I would come home to my parents arguing, screaming, and yelling. Some days, I would become so frustrated that I wouldn't go home. I would go to my best friend's house nearby for some peace, or I would submerge myself in extracurricular activities and education after school.

In late middle school, I realized my passion for the sciences and knew I wanted to become a physician to help others. My passion for helping others and giving back was evident at a very young age. I volunteered as a tutor at local elementary schools and also became a mentor to the younger girls. My teachers always considered me "an old soul" who was very wise for my young age.

Unfortunately, one autumn day in October, my life changed forever. A family that was once thought of as "picture perfect" by those on the outside was shattered. I came home from high school that Friday, wearing my favorite pair of Guess jeans, white tee, and all-white Nike Air Force Ones. As I began walking up my driveway, I could smell the scent of my mother's cooking. A smile hit my face as I immediately knew we were having smothered pork chops, collard greens, mac and cheese, and homemade buttermilk biscuits—one of my favorite meals prepared by my mother. As I walked inside our home, gospel music was blaring on the radio. I walked into the kitchen to see my mom in tears, wiping her face.

After sitting with my mom that day and having a candid conversation, even at the tender age of sixteen, I could sense the fear in my mother's eyes. I found out about a lot of things I never knew existed. The unhappiness, betrayal, and lies that she had been experiencing. I realized that my mother had been in a marriage that seemed so happy and vibrant, yet she was so alone. My parents had made the decision to separate. The news hit me like a ton of bricks, especially because in the last month, three of my friends found out their parents were going through divorces as well.

Many changes began to happen around my home during that time. My mother exemplified what I felt was the "real-life" version of what the Bible says is a virtuous woman.

My mother was a stay-at-home mom and made many sacrifices to be there for us during a time in which crime and drugs ran rampant in our city. She always wanted the best for us and did everything she could to give us the best life possible. My mother raised us rich in love (rather than money), which is priceless. Raising three kids as a single mother is not easy, but somehow my mom managed to do it through God's grace and her strength.

Because my mother was a full-time, stay-at-home mom, she had never carved out enough time for herself or to pursue her dreams. My mother always wanted to be there for our family and made sure that a parent figure was always there for support. Family time was important to my mother, and she always had activities for my brothers and me to do with her during the weekends. I enjoyed cooking with her every week and going to church every Sunday. The combination of strong core family values, prayer, and love was a strong foundation for our family and very important to my mother.

Who would have thought the legacy, strength, and vision that I saw through my mother would become my own catalyst to be the best mom I can be to my daughter? At that tender age, when I felt like my world was crashing, I did not know I would somehow come to the realization of the "why" in my thirties—almost decades later. Now, being a single mom, I know the heartache, pain, struggles, strength, and courage it takes to raise a child on your own. Learning to balance work and mothering is the biggest challenge I have ever faced in my life. When your own daughter tells her teachers, "I love my mommy, but she's always working," it is heartbreaking. I am doing everything I can to build a life for her and a legacy, yet at the ripe age of three, she is too young to comprehend the possibilities of it all. However, these days I am more motivated than ever before to be that strong role model for my daughter, like my mother was to me all those years.

I am still trying to balance this thing called life, but God is truly amazing. Currently, I am a well-known board-certified pediatrician, mother, bestselling author, consultant, speaker, and media expert. However, if it were not for my life circumstances, I would not have pushed myself to be the best, strive harder, and be persistent and driven in everything that I pursued in life. I had to learn to turn my burdens into my blessings. Through my faith in God, a strong and prayerful mother, and my prayers for my purpose-driven life, I have achieved my goals and have many more to achieve.

In today's world, it's not easy being a mom and a wife while maintaining work-life balance. Being a single mom to a child with a chronic illness has pushed me not only to provide better quality natural healthcare to my daughter through my education as a pediatrician, but I am also a guide for many mothers out there "just like me." I am not only an advocate for my child, but for all mothers.

Chapter 5

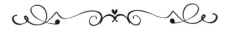

The SisFriend Saga

Dr. Teriya Richmond

As iron sharpens iron, so one person sharpens another.

Psalm 21:17

Dagnabit! I made the honor roll! It was a warm sunny day in Chicago. The breeze was magnificent, like Chicago fall weather can inconsistently be. The weather meant I could go home and be a Westsider. If you are from Chicago, you know what that insinuates. I wouldn't have rather grown up on any other side of the CHI! See, being a Westsider meant we stayed outside, whether sitting on the porch, walking to the corner store, or meeting up with our friends on the block. Our style would be considered country and sometimes a little "ghetto," if that's a description of a group of people with a unique swag and expression of oneself. Anyway, we always knew the Westside was the best side.

That day, I raced home from the bus drop-off site to do just that—meet up with my friends and share the good news. Everyone was sure to be outside already because my brothers and I were bussed to and from Walt Disney Magnet School, which was very far from home. In fact, it was located across the street from Lake Michigan, or what we affectionately call "the lakefront," on Marine Drive. Momma had been accused of being bougie—whatever that means—but she wouldn't settle for anything less for us. I stay dressed to the nines on a budget that was as quiet as it was kept. My pink and purple outfit was purchased from Madigans, Sears, Montgomery Wards, or JCPenney. I know it was one of those because they were the main stores where we shopped at North Riverside Mall.

Momma never accepted anything less than keeping my brothers and I well kept and with good—no, excellent—grades. Shoot, if I got one B with the rest all As, she would ask, what about this B, Teriya? She was always encouraging me to focus on books before boys. I didn't get that at first because, innately, I put books before boys. Man, I loved to read book after book after book. Momma would catch me reading with a small flashlight under the covers, way past my bedtime. *Are You There God? It's Me, Margaret* is one of my favorite books. I read that book over and over again.

Margaret and I had nothing in common other than being tall with long hair. She was white. I was black. Her mom and dad were married and in the same household. Anyway, I guess you could say Margaret and I were best friends. I learned what puberty and menstruation were from when Margaret got her cycle in the book. I spent more time reading about her instead of learning how to jump rope. And no, I do not know how to jump Double Dutch. But I can turn rope. When I woke up in the middle of the night at nine years old with soiled underwear, my brain said, "Remember what happened to your best friend, Margaret?"

The point is, I loved to read, learn, and get good grades. I was proud of my grades because I worked hard to get them. Certainly, my best friend since we were three years old would be happy for me. I knew she could see me happily skipping up the street with some good news to share. She was smiling.

"Shawn, I got all As!"

BOP! Came the first lick.

BOP! Came the second lick.

Hold on! Hold on! Hold on! My mind was not understanding at all. What did I do? I'd just gotten home from school. I looked up to you, I thought to myself. I literally begged Momma to let me get my hair like yours. Those French braids with the multicolored beads at the end were it to me. But not to Momma. She said that the hairstyle is not healthy for your hair. Perhaps her refusal to let me copy your hair was a prelude to what she really meant. She meant I was different.

I was thinking, how did my sharing my good grades turn into her basically kicking my butt? The truth was, Momma was right. I was different, special, and unique. So I knew this was the aloha—yes, the hello and goodbye—of that "friendship." But deep down inside, I hoped not. I thought, I cannot tell Momma about this. She would never let me hang with her again, and I would be stuck with Margaret.

The trouble was that Margaret was in a book, but this was no fairy tale.

I did tell Momma but only the partial truth. The best thing to do was tell her my friend was not happy for me when I shared my good news, but I was never ever going to tell her the girl put her hands on me.

Apparently, my heart yearned for connections with sisfriends, as I liked to call them, to my own detriment. I continued the relationship with Shawn, albeit differently, but as a preteen, my life revolved around friends. I suppose that was common for preteens and teenagers. I went hard for all of my friends, perhaps because I did not grow up with any sisters. There was me and my two brothers, and then three more boy cousins until they moved. Somehow, I would hold on to "friends" who meant me no good. It has been my pattern from day one. You would think I would have figured it out, but I didn't. I wanted to stay sisfriends with all my sisfriends for life, but I realized some sisfriends are in my life for a reason and a season, and only a few are meant to be there for a lifetime.

High school was fun. My friends and I hung out like we were in college. By this time, I worked three jobs and was paying for most of my luxuries. One night, my girls and I were getting ready for the club. I called one of my friends and asked, "Girl, what you wearing?"

Her response was, "Nothing, some jeans and a tee shirt."

I showed up and my sisfriends were in leather and fur. I thought we had a consensus on jeans and tee shirts. Perhaps they had forgotten to call and let me know the cohesive dress code had changed. But on the other hand, maybe that was intentional. Of course, that never came to mind. Not that it mattered what we were wearing, but in the moment, I just wanted to be friends and to be liked so badly that I continued the relationships.

Growing up out West (yes, the Westside of Chicago), no one was talking about going to medical school or even college for that matter, other than if they were asking me, girl, why you want to do that? Oh, you the college girl, huh? Most of the time, these questions were asked with a negative connotation, but I never thought it was the reality. Then a light bulb went off. I still considered myself the victim and was trying to figure out why the sisfriends who I held so dearly to my heart would then turn around and stomp on it. But more importantly, what was it about me that allowed it to happen?

To answer this question, I had to do some introspection. This habit of subjecting myself to relationships that looked great on the outside, or seemed like the sisfriend had my best interest at heart but not really, was a puzzle that needed to be figured out. I love super hard—even before I know if the love is reciprocated. I give freely even if I don't know if it will be given back.

Growing up, I did everything I could to please my mother and make her proud. I know she is well pleased with me now. However, growing up, I thought she wanted me to be perfect. She really just wanted me to be the best me I could be. God had given me a gift, a gift of being able to love my "sisters" unconditionally. I just hadn't learned how to protect that gift and to protect my heart. Yes, indeed, every time I played the victim. I kept thinking, why me? Well, why not me? My experiences over time and growth helped me to change my mindset. I decided to not be a victim but a victor. I pledged that I would be an overcomer!

I took a few steps to get this "sisterhood" thing right. These steps are in no particular order:

Step #1: Do a little introspection. Look back on your childhood and relationships with your parents and family members. Ask God to reveal how those interactions play into your mindset as an adult.

Step #2: List your motives. Are you seeking relationships just to please others or to get what you can out of another sister? Is your attraction to that person due to external or superficial qualities?

Step #3: When you see the first signs of an unhealthy, unrequited relationship, try to determine if the relationship is really meant for a reason, season, or lifetime.

Step #4: Pray. Pray. Pray.

Step #5: If the "sistership" is only for a reason or season and not a lifetime, "LIG" it! Let it go!

Chapter 6

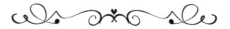

A Blessing in Disguise

Damaria Edwards

*Behold, children are a heritage from the Lord,
the fruit of the womb a reward.*

Psalm 127:3-5 (ESV)

After only three short years of marriage, I felt legally married but emotionally single. I had no idea how I had lost myself in the marriage and had fallen out of love with the man I vowed before God to spend the rest of my life with. What had gone wrong? Why did my marriage feel like a chore? I was tired of putting in so much energy and getting nothing in return. It wasn't that my husband didn't love me or that he treated me badly. On the surface, we were this young black power couple who others looked up to, but emotionally, I felt disconnected from him and unsure of what I even enjoyed outside of the marriage.

To add insult to injury, our sex life had completely gone down the drain with no hope for recovery. When I would voice my frustration to my older friends, many of them would say sex isn't everything, which I completely agreed with, but at twenty-eight years old, I was in my prime, and it didn't seem fair not to be able to have great sex with my husband so early on in the marriage.

Financially, we were comfortable. I had recently become a nurse, and my husband had received a promotion at his job, but the hours created an even bigger wedge between us than I wanted to openly admit. We had a beautiful apartment in the 'burbs, and most importantly, our two boys, who were eight and nine years old at the time, were happy and healthy. In the beginning of our relationship, my husband and I would do everything together, and after getting married, we tried our best to continue to go on a date at least once a month, which seemed reasonable at the time with two kids under the age of ten. However, as we grew, so did the space between us. I started questioning, what had I truly signed up for? Who was this man I married? Who was I? Is this really what marriage is about? I slowly stopped praying for my marriage and eventually lost all hope in it. Instead of seeking counseling or continuing to pray for my marriage, I found another man who could fill the void in my marriage.

The affair started out as just occasional sex, but as it carried on for several months, the frequency of our visits increased from once a week to three to four times a week. We would talk for hours about our goals and dreams, places we wanted to visit, and things we wanted from our significant others, and I felt free to be myself without judgment, which was a big issue in my marriage.

This man and I both worked the night shift, while my husband worked an odd night or early morning shift, which didn't allow for us to spend much time together. When my husband was awake, I was asleep and vice versa. This left a huge window of opportunity to be with the other man while my kids were at school. I let this man into a personal space that I had not let my husband into, and I couldn't understand how that had happened. I had been with my husband since I was nineteen years old, so he was really the only man I had been with as an adult. But now that I was twenty-eight years old and no longer desired my husband's direction, it felt more like him telling me what and how to do things versus advising me on a better way to do things. I had become resentful. After much contemplation, I decided it was best to walk away from the affair before things got too carried away, but I think the decision was a little too late.

After feelings of guilt weighed me down and out of the desire to reconcile, I confessed to my husband about the affair. He said deep down he already knew something wasn't right between us, but we decided to work on the marriage and move forward. To spice up our sex life, my husband and I started to experiment with different sex toys and have sex in random places. We started dating intentionally, without the distractions of electronics, to rekindle the connection we had clearly lost.

Six weeks later, I realized I had missed my menstrual cycle, so I took a pregnancy test. It only confirmed what I knew in my gut. My husband was excited about having another child. I was devastated because I was unsure of who the father was and if I should keep the child I was carrying. I thought to myself, what have I done? How could I have been so careless? What do I do now? Should I bring another life into this world with all this confusion involved? Was this really the path God wanted me to take, or had I gotten so far off course that I didn't know what direction I was going in? Would I be able to overcome this state of confusion?

I cried for several days while trying to hold everything together and carry on with my everyday life as if nothing had happened—until one day, I came to work to take care of a patient like I normally would and ended up crying the entire day. The inability to control my tears made me realize I had reached the lowest point in my life. I didn't know what to do next.

I had made up my mind and called the abortion clinic to make an appointment. I thought this would fix everything and I could carry on with my life. But then I thought, would it really fix anything? My husband insisted we keep the child even though he had no idea what we were about to take on by brushing this major secret under the rug. God sent a praying friend my way to help shield me from the verbal backlash that would soon come, but also to guide me to a life coach, a non-biased person who could help me pick up the pieces of my crumbling life.

My first session with the life coach was supposed to be two hours, but it turned into four hours. It was a turning point in my life. We talked about my past experiences, or as she referred to them, footprints, that mold you as a child and greatly affect your actions and decisions as an adult; my present, which consisted of a broken marriage and uncertainty about the father of the unborn child in my womb; and my future and what I wanted to change.

I cried my heart out because I had lost love for myself and was beyond a state of confusion. My life coach prayed with me and for my unborn king. The very next day after the meeting, I called the abortion clinic and canceled the appointment. That is one of the best decisions I have ever made, despite all the storms that came along with that journey.

Of course, that was only the beginning of a long journey to restore the woman of God I am today. I met with my life coach on a weekly basis, and we would discuss every aspect of my life, my relationship with my mother and sisters, the life-changing experiences I had endured as a child, and my circle of friends. She gave me different tips to help me regain self-love and forgiveness. I felt like I was on the right track to restore my faith and peace of mind. My husband was as supportive as he could be throughout the entire pregnancy, even though we hadn't fully healed from the infidelity that we had committed (yes, my husband had cheated too). But now we were bringing a life into the world and we were going to do our best to push through the trials and tribulations.

Once the baby arrived, things went downhill. I had convinced myself the baby was my husband's and as long as neither of the two potential fathers mentioned a DNA test, then I wasn't going to bring it up, even though I had assured my husband that we could take a DNA test when the baby arrived if he wanted to, but he said it was not necessary. Although my husband didn't mention the DNA test, he felt the baby looked nothing like him and started to question if his parents had pictures of himself when he was a child. The elephant in the room grew because of the lack of discussion about who the biological father of the child was, postpartum depression had fully kicked in, and I was unsure of how to deal with the struggles. I couldn't afford to see the life coach anymore, and with a newborn, getting out of the house was even more of a struggle, so I put on a smile and carried on with my life. Deep down inside, we were not okay at all.

We attended married couple events and retreats but never asked for help with the issues we had because that meant we had to admit to our sins and weaknesses. Both our parents did not have successful marriages, and I was his second wife, so we didn't have good examples in our inner circle. Many of our married friends were having issues as well. We tried to stay strong, but once the results of the DNA test came back, the marriage ended shortly thereafter.

I started dating the man I cheated with shortly after I left my husband, and within two months, I was pregnant again. Not only had I not given myself time to heal from the ending of my marriage, but I had started a whole new family without truly dating this man. It sent me into a downhill spiral that I felt compelled to deal with because I had made my bed and I needed to lie in it. I loved him, but at that time in my life, I needed to love myself more than anyone else besides God. I cried and complained about things that really shouldn't have been an issue. I was very impatient and easily frustrated with situations. It was even harder to date him with a one-year-old and being pregnant, so we were at a standstill even though he was trying to adjust to me and the emotional roller coaster I was on.

For almost six months, I hid the pregnancy from people who weren't in my inner circle and didn't talk to many people before I openly admitted I was having another child. My best friend and I were pregnant at the same time, but while she was excited to be having another baby with her husband, I was depressed about having another child. Once my fourth son was born, on my father's birthday, I was filled with a temporary joy, but little did I know the depression would soon reach an all-time high.

My newborn and I cried almost every day for no reason; plus my boyfriend and I argued a lot over small things. I started praying and asked God to remove this terrible mental disease that was taking over my life. Once I went back to work after being off for three months, I started to feel some relief from the daily crying, but I was far from healed. I had to openly admit I was depressed, so I could truly get some help. I saw a counselor, continued to pray, and found a church I looked forward to going to. It took me almost two years to truly overcome the long battle to forgive myself for the infidelity, the child outside of marriage, the failed marriage, and the almost failed relationship with my two youngest kids' father. Despite the ups and downs, he has truly stood by me even when I have walked away from him.

Today, I can say I have forgiven myself for the mistakes I have made, the confusion I have caused, and the guilt I have carried, and I would not change any of my trials or tribulations because they have made me a stronger and wiser woman of God. I believe there is life after divorce, and I love my four boys so much—they are the reason I am still standing.

Here are three takeaways from my testimony:

When you go through difficult times in your life, don't give up! The trials and tribulations you overcome in life will become your testimony and ultimately be a blessing to someone else.

Don't suffer in any situation in silence. Most people don't share their story or even ask for help during a storm because they are in fear of what others will think. Only God can judge you! Evaluate your circle, remove negative people, and surround yourself with positive, uplifting people who will help you no matter what direction life takes you.

Men are not the only ones who have babies outside of their marriage. I am not condoning infidelity by any means, but the reality is it happens a lot more than people are willing to admit. If and when it does, you either stand by your mate during the storm or separate for your own peace of mind; but understand that there is life after both decisions, and don't allow anyone to make your sin hold yourself back from moving forward in life.

Chapter 7

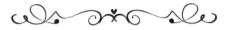

You Can't Steal My Joy

Shanicka N. Scarbrough, MD

For our struggle is not against flesh and blood, but against the rulers, against the authorities, against the powers of this dark world and against the spiritual forces of evil in the heavenly realms.

Ephesians 6:12 (NIV)

I had returned home from school on a regular afternoon. My grandmother used to keep me until my mother came home late in the evenings, after a long day of work. I was ten years old at the time, and like any other preteen, I would try to test my limits with how sassy my mouth could be without being backhanded. I tried it with my grandmother that day, running my big mouth as usual. She was just outdone by my brazen disrespect, and instead of reprimanding me or, thankfully, putting her hands on me, she called my mother at work. Now, every black child knows that if it goes that far as to disturb your parent at work, you are definitely in for "it." My grandmother handed me the phone, and I heard the words that struck fear into my core being: "You just wait until I get home." I knew what that meant. I would get the black beat off of me!

Most children would simply tremble in fear, be on their best behavior for the rest of the evening, or create an "I'm sorry" card or treat—anything to avoid the butt whooping that they knew was on the way. This was usually my modus operandi, but for some reason, I thought it was a better idea to simply take myself out of the equation completely. I went into my grandmother's medicine cabinet, grabbed a bottle of acetaminophen, and with a glass of orange juice, downed as many as I could. At the time, I was not depressed nor had I experienced previous thoughts of self-mutilation or suicide. I am not even sure if I knew what suicide meant. The one thing that I did know was that I didn't want to be there by the time my mother got home.

Everything after that was a blur of flashing lights and a feeling of weariness in my soul. Then I was sitting in a hospital bed, a plastic object in my mouth so that I wouldn't bite down on the hose that was being shoved down my throat. Into my stomach, they were pumping what I know now to be activated charcoal to counter the effects of the acetaminophen. I'll never forget the thick black substance that was being pumped into my stomach that eventually came back out via my stool and vomit. I thought I would never do anything so stupid again. The tears and pure terror in my mother and grandmother's eyes as they looked down on me should have thwarted any inkling of a thought of this happening again, but when the devil has it out for you, he will stop at nothing to destroy you.

That was not the last time I tried to commit suicide. The next time, I was fourteen years old, a freshman in high school. It happened one evening after seemingly a regular day of school work and after-school activities. I was lying on the floor of my bedroom, with the phone cradled between my shoulder and chin, talking on a three-way call with two of my best friends. Complete sadness washed over me, and while I was chatting with them about nothing, I began to take those same pills that I had taken just four years prior. As I became drowsy, I began to cry, alerting my friends that something was wrong. They were finally able to get it out of me that I had taken pills to "go to sleep for good."

My girlfriends quickly jumped into action and contacted my mother, who was cooking in the other room, and I was rushed to the hospital. I don't have any recollection of that hospital stay, but I do recall being sent home with no further treatment given. In retrospect, there should have been more of a push for me to get the help that I so desperately needed, but as all things mental go, it was swept under the rug by my treating physician and by my family.

The whole ordeal was baffling to myself and my family. I did not have an unhappy childhood. I had not experienced any traumatic events in my life. My mother and I had a healthy dose of teenager-against-mom-and-the-world in our relationship, but nothing that would trigger such dramatic responses to what is seemingly the life of the average black child. I did not grow up in poverty, I had many friends and acquaintances, I was very active in extracurricular activities, and I was an honor student. I was outgoing and had a cheery disposition around those I came in contact with. I could not put my finger on any reason why, on occasion, I would feel an indescribable feeling of emptiness, longing, and despair.

It would be almost ten years before I would try to take my life again, but over the course of those years, I would spiral in and out of a depressive state, with various circumstances driving me deeper and closer to self-destruction. My sadness would lead to poor decisions with resultant consequences that would make it harder to feel like life could get any better. It was a vicious cycle of drowning in self-pity and despair, creating ripples and then waves of unfortunate and often avoidable situations. My mind was clouded. I had difficulty adjusting to the many aspects that make up a life, which impaired my ability to have healthy relationships with colleagues, friends, and even family. I found myself in and out of the hospital for severe depression, and I was diagnosed with bipolar disorder. I was placed on a multitude of medications with the aim of stabilizing my mood, in addition to weekly therapy. I was not in a good place and, despite all of the treatment modalities in place, I did not know how to come out of it.

I had grown up in the church but did not truly understand its purpose. And interestingly, I had accepted Christ at a young age, around the age of eight, just two years before my first suicide attempt. I asked Jesus to come into my heart and I felt my heart thump in my chest. As I think back on it, I believe that was God's way of showing my young self that He heard my request and was truly with me. But it wasn't until it felt like my mind completely snapped and I was truly at the lowest place I could have ever imagined to be, that I was able to call on His name for help. I knew that this was not how I wanted to spend the rest of my life. The doctors couldn't fix me, self-help books weren't doing it, and conversations with my friends and family were not helping.

As a last resort, during the pivotal shift between my twenties and my thirties, I cried out to God, asking Him to take this burden from me. I didn't want to feel like this anymore. I did not want to continue hurting myself and others. I needed something bigger and greater than me to step in and change me from the inside out.

I can tell you with certainty that in that instance, I felt a literal weight being lifted from me. Psalm 34:17 (NIV) says, "The righteous cry out, and the LORD hears them; he delivers them from all their troubles." I began to go back to church, read the word for myself, and develop a relationship with Christ. I learned things from scriptures that encouraged me and helped me see the truth, the real reason behind my sadness, self-loathing, and self-destructive behavior. All of those years, Satan was whispering suggestions in my ear that I was not worthy, that I was a failure, that I didn't deserve love, and that I deserved to die. The devil is a liar! I would always hear this statement, but it really began to ring true for me once I recommitted myself to Christ, and His word revealed the wonderful truths of God's love and His will on my life. John 10:10 says, "The thief [the devil] comes only to steal and kill and destroy; I [God] have come that they may have life, and have it to the full." What good news!

My life changed when everything I thought I knew was reshaped by how God viewed me. You see, the devil knows that if you believe in Christ and all of His promises, and if you develop your own relationship with Him and begin to tap into your full potential, therefore discovering God's will on your life, you will be unstoppable and wreak havoc on the devil's plans to destroy you. He doesn't want you to be armed with the truth. He wants to keep you shackled. He doesn't want your life to change, he doesn't want to see your change affect those around you, and he doesn't want you to impact the world by leading others to Christ. He knows that true change is infectious, and your light will shine so that others will see God through you and your life. But John 8:36 reminds us that "if the Son sets you free, you will be free indeed."

The last time I suffered from depression and was delivered from the diagnosis of bipolar disorder was in 2009. I have not taken a mood stabilizer, antipsychotic, or antidepressant since that time! My joy comes from the Lord, and my light is shining bright as the Holy Spirit continues to work on and through me. Romans 15:13 says, "May the God of hope fill you with all joy and peace as you trust in him, so that you may overflow with hope by the power of the Holy Spirit."

The key to this whole shebang is to *trust in Him*! This, I know, can initially be no easy task. This didn't happen overnight for me. God had to perform some true miracles in my life for me to begin to actively trust in His word. As God continued to show his love for me, I became more willing to accept his love and even more willing to reject the lies that the devil was so apt to whisper in my ear. I began to live out James 4:7, which says, "Submit yourselves, then, to God. Resist the devil, and he will flee from you." And then I watched my life take a drastic turn toward peace of mind and spirit.

This is not to say that my life since then has been free of problems. Life is a daily struggle of complicated circumstances, mishaps, and the challenge of interacting with people who know and love Christ in their various levels of spiritual maturity, as well as those who do not know Him at all. The difference now is how I respond to them and my problems and struggles. I no longer allow my problems to define who I am. I no longer allow emotions to rule my decisions. I try to approach each situation with a clear mind and heart and take it to God in search of a divine answer to my questions. I am not always successful, but I am quickly reminded how hard it is to try to handle life with my own strength and end up having to return to my Father for answers. I am now armed with the knowledge that I have a choice about how I interact with my environment. I can choose to be led by the Holy Spirit and be victorious over any situation or emotion, including depression. You see, God has given us free will. It's what we do with it that matters. We cannot control our circumstances, but we can control our emotions and our reactions to them. It feels so much better to let go of the things that were oppressing me, and walk boldly in faith and trust in God's promises.

I share my story with you because I want you to know that there is a life of abundance waiting for you, if you would only make the decision to choose Christ. I do not promise that life will not have its ups and downs, and I do not promise that if you accept Christ today or even if you are a devout Christian, that tomorrow your life will be filled with roses and sunshine. But I can promise you that your life will change. I will promise you that if you continue to walk and grow with Christ that you can defeat the demons that plague your life as they plagued mine. I can guarantee that if you seek Him first, your purpose and will on your life will be revealed, giving you direction and guidance on how you can do your part to build the kingdom. I know that these are bold promises, but I can only speak from a place of experience and deliverance.

I now know how I was attacked in an effort to thwart me from my God-given destiny, even at a very young age, with the sole goal of preventing me from sharing the good news that God loves each and every one of us. The devil does not fight fair, but the good news is that he can be and is defeated! God is calling us to be the salt of the earth and the light of the world (Matthew 5:13-16) so that others may see the goodness of Christ through our deeds and in turn glorify Him. Not a bad deal if you ask me! This is my prayer; perhaps it can be yours too:

> *Lord, I believe in you. I believe that Christ died on the cross for my sins. Come into my heart so that my life can be forever changed. Guide my steps and connect me with people who serve you and glorify your name, that I might grow spiritually and have the strength and courage, through my own testimony of victory and deliverance, to bear much fruit. I know my problems are not bigger than you and I release them all to you. Heal me, comfort me, guide*

me, love me. Remove anything that is not like you from my mind, body, and spirit, and I will give you all of the praise and glory. It's in the mighty name of Jesus I pray, Amen.

Author's Corner

LACHELLE EVANS

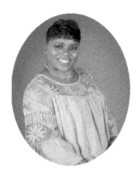

Born in Chicago, Illinois, Lachelle Evans is a mother of four young adults, glam-mother of five, and care assistant to her mother. With over twenty years of customer service experience, Lachelle currently works as a customer service representative for the Chicago Transit Authority (CTA). She hopes to open a nonprofit organization entitled IMEE to **i**nspire, **m**entor, **e**mpower, and **e**ncourage men, women, boys, and girls, of all ages and races.

Having grown up in church and developed a strong love for God, Lachelle loves telling everyone she meets how blessed and fabulous they are, and she has a passion for helping others with her big golden smile. As a newlywed, she enjoys spending time with the love of her life, family, and friends. She also enjoys cooking, shopping, traveling, and trying new things.

Timika Lucas

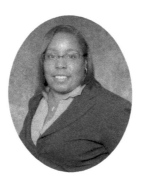

Born and raised in Chicago, Illinois, Timika Lucas is the oldest of three girls. Her love of helping others motivated her to work in healthcare, where she currently serves as a reimbursement specialist. Timika earned her bachelor's degree in health administration and a master's degree with a concentration in health services.

After delivering her third child prematurely, Timika wants to help others who have gone or are going through the same experience. She is in the process of growing her business, Lucas RCM Consultants, which teaches physicians about revenue cycle management (RCM). Timika resides in the south suburbs of Chicago with her husband and three children.

To connect, visit her website at
www.lucasrcmconsultants.com

Dr. Jerisa Berry

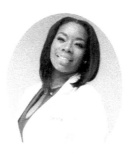

As one of the nation's acclaimed doctors, Dr. Jerisa Berry, aka Dr. Jerisa ER, is a nationally recognized speaker, media consultant, and author. Board-certified in emergency medicine, she is on staff at several emergency facilities in South Florida and, with her husband, is the co-owner of Vital Care Medical Center, Inc. Dr. Jerisa is also the founder of SecureYourFertility.com, where she helps single ladies and career-minded women take control of their fertility.

After graduating from Howard University, Dr. Jerisa earned her medical degree from New York College of Osteopathic Medicine, and completed her internship and dual residency in emergency medicine and family medicine at Midwestern University. When she is not saving lives in the ER, as a sought-after media expert, Dr. Jerisa shares her expertise in real-world health strategies regarding acute, emergent, and chronic health conditions.

Dr. Tamika Bush

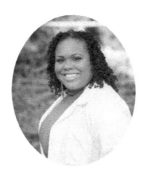

Dr. Tamika Bush, DO (Dr. TamikaPeds), is a highly respected and well-known board-certified pediatrician and doctor mom. An expert on children's health and natural ways to keep children healthy without the use of conventional medicine, Dr. Bush dedicates her professional career to helping children any way she can through her vast knowledge of pediatric medicine

Dr. Bush earned her doctor of osteopathic medicine from Kansas City University of Medicine and Biosciences and completed her pediatric training at St. John Hospital and Medical Center. Dr. Bush is a Fellow of the American Academy of Pediatrics and proud member of The American College of Osteopathic Pediatricians. In her spare time, Dr. Bush enjoys spending time with her daughter and family.

To connect, visit her website at
www.drtamikapeds.com

DR. TERIYA RICHMOND

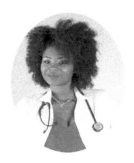

Teriya Monick Richmond was born and raised in Chicago, Illinois. After attending Mount Saint College in Clinton, Iowa, Dr. Richmond continued her education at the University of Illinois College of Medicine and School of Public Health, where she received her master of public health and doctor of medicine.

Dr. Richmond is committed to bringing quality, evidence-based medical care to the minority community and has a passion for women's health issues. Currently, she provides patient care to uninsured and underinsured patients at Acres Home Health Center and LBJ hospital, and in February 2017, Dr. Richmond opened her own health services clinic.

Dr. Richmond and her husband of eight years, Jack, are parents to four-year-old son, Jaxon.

To connect, email her at
mochmilw@gmail.com

Damaria Anderson-Edwards

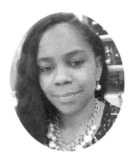

Damaria Anderson-Edwards, also known as "Sweet Dee," is a licensed practical nurse who also runs a small meal-prepping business called Healthy Eats by Sweet Dee. Damaria has a passion for helping people and living a healthy lifestyle. Her favorite scripture from the Bible is Philippians 4:13: "I can do all things through Christ who strengthens me."

A mother to four boys, Damaria enjoys taking walks, skating, and bike riding. In the near future, she plans to open a health and wellness center, which will have a holistic approach for living a healthy lifestyle mentally and physically, as well as go back to school to further her career in the healthcare field.

To connect, email Damaria at
sweetdeehealthyeats@gmail.com

SHANICKA N. SCARBROUGH, MD

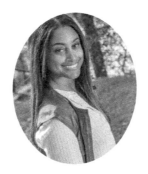

Dr. Shanicka Scarbrough (aka America's Favorite Family Doctor) graduated from the University of Illinois College of Medicine in 2009 and completed her family medicine residency program at Advocate Christ Medical Center in 2012. Since then, she has gained invaluable experience as a board-certified family medicine physician and has had the privilege of owning and operating a private medical practice. She now teaches other physicians and physicians-in-training how to start their own medical practice with her bestselling book, *The Lunchtime Physician Entrepreneur*, and her live virtual courses in the Road to Private Practice Academy.

Dr. Shanicka's mission is to be transparent about her life in hopes that sharing her testimonies will help bring others closer to God. Having hosted the The DivaMD radio show on Urban Broadcast Media, and continuing to contribute to a variety of other platforms on television and social media, she speaks in various educational settings and travels internationally, including to Haiti and South Africa, to extend her knowledge, skills, and expertise across the globe.

To connect, visit her website at

www.DrShanicka.com

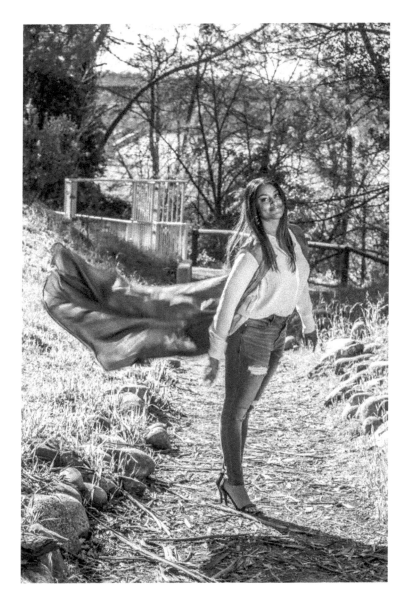

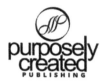

CREATING DISTINCTIVE BOOKS
WITH INTENTIONAL RESULTS

We're a collaborative group of creative masterminds
with a mission to produce high-quality books to position
you for monumental success in the marketplace.

Our professional team of writers, editors, designers,
and marketing strategists work closely together to ensure
that every detail of your book is a clear representation
of the message in your writing.

Want to know more?
Write to us at info@publishyourgift.com
or call (888) 949-6228

Discover great books, exclusive offers, and more at
www.PublishYourGift.com

Connect with us on social media

@publishyourgift

CPSIA information can be obtained
at www.ICGtesting.com
Printed in the USA
LVHW021112040219
606286LV00026BA/703/P